MW00933941

This notebook belongs to:

____

Made in the USA
Coppell, TX
08 March 2022

74685991R10068